A Doula's Guide
to
The Placenta

By Jemmais Keval-Baxter
The Ho'oponopono Doula™

Published by Matrilineal Ink

Matrilineal Ink

www.matrilineal.cl

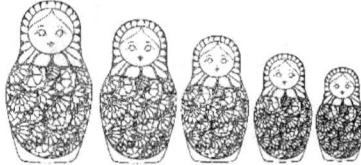

Published by: Matrilineal Ink™
www.matrilineal.cl
ISBN: 978-1-9998071-5-3

A Doula's Guide to The Placenta

By Jemmais Keval-Baxter
The Ho'oponopono Doula™

Published by Matrilineal Ink

Matrilineal Ink

www.matrilineal.cl

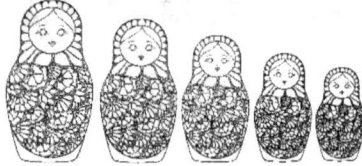

Other books in the series include:
A Doula's Guide to Education
A Doula's Guide to Nutrition
A Doula's Guide to Breastfeeding
A Doula's Guide to Menstruation

Also by Jemmais Keval-Baxter
Ho'oponopono Birth: Ho'oponopono
for Pregnancy and Childbirth

Table of Contents

Introduction

Before we take our first steps into the profound and mysterious world of pregnancy and motherhood, we rarely have the opportunity to consider the existence of the placenta. The placenta accompanies all of us during our time in the womb, our first companion, our constant and ever faithful friend and protector, yet, many us do not know what happened to ours, and we have probably never thought to ask.

Childbirth is a rite of passage, a significant initiation into motherhood that preparation for it often takes up a great deal of our time, we prepare for the birth and the arrival of our new baby's, yet the birth of the placenta, the afterbirth, is usually an afterthought.

In this short guide, I hope to introduce some of the wonders of the placenta, acquaint you with the ways it helps to nurture and care for our unborn children. I will present traditional beliefs around honoring the placenta and even delve into the latest trend of consuming the placenta in tinctures, capsule, and smoothies as a reported healing aid.

What is the Placenta?

"The placenta is the first mother to each of us. It feeds us and is there for us, providing all we need to grow. The placenta is our sustainer and protector, our first love felt in the body, the first experience of unconditional love we receive. When we are cut-off from this first source of love prematurely, it leads to us seeking love outside of our own self, in a conditional way. Sadly, this is what happens to more than 99 percent of us when our umbilical cord is prematurely cut when we are born ... from our life force and soul connection, which is still pulsing through the cord connecting us to the placenta. This cut happens before the placenta has transferred its emotional nurturing qualities and soul essence to us. This sudden separation creates shock and fear, borne out of ignorance for the deeper connection between life, love, mother, and child."[1.]

The placenta is both an organ and a gland, its functions are multiple. First, the placenta is responsible for producing hormones which encourage the growth of the fetus it supplies estrogen, progesterone, somatomammotropin and human placental lactogen which helps to maintain the mother's pregnancy and prepare her for breastfeeding after the birth.

In addition to producing hormones, the placenta also acts as a protective barrier between the mother and the child, ensuring that the circulatory systems of each are kept separate. This is vital as it provides protection to the fetus from many toxins and bacterial infections that could affect the mother.

If there are any abnormalities in the mother's blood, the placenta acts as a protective barrier for the embryo. Although some viral infections can pass through the placenta. In some cases, the placenta is even capable of protecting a child from a severe disease such as HIV, which may affect the mother but not her child. (The World Health Organization recommends that all HIV positive pregnant and breastfeeding women and their infants should receive appropriate antiretroviral (ARV) drugs to prevent mother to child transmission of HIV.)

The placenta is formed from the same union of sperm and egg as the fetus, growing alongside the child and implanting into the uterine wall of the mother. Indonesian cultures regard the placenta as the spiritual twin of the child and take great care to honor the placenta after birth. They believe that the spirit of the child must be reunited with its twin or elder sibling (the placenta) before journeying on to the afterlife, or risk walking the earth as a ghost in search of its nurturing companion.

"In many sacred traditions, the placenta is seen as our twin soul, our double ... a second child, the child's double, with the placenta also having its own soul that resides in the umbilical cord. Ancient Egyptian Pharaohs believed one soul inhabited the body, and the other the placenta, with the placenta respected and honored as their guardian, and as their twin from birth; a valued part of themselves, not separate or useless.... I feel my placenta is my own connection to the love of the universe and a divine connection to other human beings. It's my first connection to universal, unconditional love.... In Cambodia the placenta is known as "the globe of the origin of the soul," and for the Maori, it is the whenua (the land) that nourishes the

people... Mother, child, and land are all intimately interconnected, each nourishing and sustaining the other. "[1.]

"Some Native Americans dried the umbilical cord, then strung it with beads, the child wore it as a talisman and was encouraged to chew on it when teething...... In parts of Malaysia and Africa, the afterbirth is viewed as either a younger or older sibling of the child. It's wrapped and buried ceremonially, in the belief that the two will be reunited after death." [2.]

The placenta is very nurturing. It is joined to the child via the umbilical cord and provides all the oxygen, nutrients, and fluid that a baby needs as well as carrying away all waste products. The attachment of the umbilical cord to the placenta, from the baby's side, resembles the tributary branching of a river or a tree and has been described as the original tree of life.

After the first 10 weeks of gestation, the placenta is fully functional, and its powerful protection is the reason that most pregnancies are considered less vulnerable after the first trimester.

Identical twins share a single placenta, which grows from the same original cells that they do. However fraternal twins (that is non-identical twins formed from separate fertilized eggs) each have their own placenta.

Placenta Previa and Placenta Accreta

The place of attachment of the placenta to the mother's uterus is vital for ensuring the safety of the pregnancy. If the placenta implants too low down in the womb then it could cause a problem, covering or partially covering the opening of the uterus where the child would naturally be born, this is **Placenta Previa** and is often cited as a cause for a planned cesarean section.

Even if the placenta is not so low down that it causes a barrier to vaginal birth, if it is not implanted in the optimal position, it may increase the risk of hemorrhage in the mother during or after childbirth. Some women have reported migration of the placenta to a higher position through a dedicated regime of visualization, positive affirmations and inverted yoga positions, such as shoulder stands. In addition to following advice on adequate nutrition and other cleansing and purifying practices emotional, physical, mental and spiritual, that are recommended during pregnancy. Even sleeping with the foot of their bed raised. If you are hoping to avoid a cesarean, then anything is worth a try, and sincere belief can manifest miracles.

Another abnormal formation of the placenta is where the placenta's growth extends into the tissue of the mother, through her uterine wall or beyond, this is **Placenta Accreta.** Placenta Accreta can cause life-threatening complications, including premature birth, impaired growth, or stillbirth for the baby, and severe hemorrhage, hysterectomy, and even death for the mother. The rates of Placenta Accreta have risen significantly in correlation with the rates of cesarean sections, and it is more likely for a woman who has received a cesarean section in previous pregnancies to be at risk of developing this severe complication. Placental abruption (the placenta detaching too early) is another potential risk which is increased after a prior cesarean.

Placenta Accreta may require surgery. If a hysterectomy is at any point raised as a potential risk of your childbirth or pregnancy, it is advisable to request that the ovaries remain intact within the mother's body after the hysterectomy, rather than being removed with the womb. The ovaries can continue to produce female hormones for the mother throughout the rest of their cycle even if she can no longer bear children. If the ovaries are removed, then it is more likely that a woman may require artificial hormone replacements after surgery, removing the ovaries is essentially an extreme and abrupt menopause.

In the case where there is the threat of the placenta becoming detached before full term *"Midwives claim that the vitamin E glues the placenta back."* [3.]

Thankfully, these conditions are extremely rare, the risk of abnormal implantation of the placenta is seriously increased with each cesarean that is performed on a woman, this is one of many reasons to avoid elective and medically unnecessary cesareans.

Ina May Gaskin mentions in her classic natural childbirth book "Spiritual Midwifery," that some doctors were saving time by stitching up just one layer of the mother's uterus after performing a cesarean section, rather than sewing two layers. This has dramatically increased the risk of uterine rupture (which can seriously endanger the life of the mother) during subsequent pregnancies. Make sure that you have written instructions which explicitly request double layer suturing in the event of cesarean being performed on you or your wife/partner, and that you remember to mention it at the time of surgery.

Birth of the Afterbirth

Once the child is born, it is necessary for the mother to give birth to the afterbirth, the placenta. In many controlled environments, such as hospitals it is routine for nurses to administer an injection of Pitocin as the baby is recovering (possibly this would be an additional injection of Pitocin if it has already been used to induce or augment labor). If you have an IV drip attached to your arm, then medication will be supplied through the IV. Make sure that you pay attention to anyone attempting to add new medication at this time and make sure that your wishes are well known especially if you would rather not receive this injection without some indication that it is medically necessary in your case. It's always worth reminding staff as they often have so many patients to deal with at any one time that it is not fair to expect them to remember everyone's specific requirements and they may simply act out of habit.

Pitocin causes the uterus to contract and expel the placenta. Uterine contractions immediately after the birth of the baby are very important, not just to expel the placenta and any additional fluid within the womb, but also to prevent additional bleeding from the mother which can lead to hemorrhage. When the placenta is attached to the mother, it receives constant blood flow from the mother's circulation through a myriad of blood vessels. When the placenta detaches, it is the contraction of the uterine muscles that seal these blood vessels and prevent excess bleeding.

Under natural circumstances, a healthy, well-nourished woman will produce an extra burst of Oxytocin as the baby is born, which stimulates uterine contractions naturally so that she will give birth to her placenta within half an hour to one hour after the birth of her child, without any need for additional medical interventions.

Just as with childbirth, the birth of the placenta is greatly aided by gravity. Where possible and if the mother has strength, she may find it helpful to get onto her knees or into a low squat, preferably with additional support (she may feel a little shaky after the effort of birthing the baby) while she, or someone trusted, cradles the baby, close to her body, so as to avoid any tension or tearing of the umbilical cord.

Make sure to wait until the mother feels the contractions rather than trying to force the placenta out without the help of her body. Suckling by the newborn on the mother's breast will stimulate the release of Oxytocin and cause uterine contractions which help to expel the placenta.

40 Days

Even after the placenta is born, there remains a great deal of extra blood, fluids, and other materials within the womb which will be slowly cleansed over a period of about 40 days. Every time that a woman breastfeeds her child her body will produce Prolactin and Oxytocin which stimulates contractions of the uterus, expelling this excess material and helping the uterus to return to its original size. Breastfeeding over the first few weeks will likely result in the mother being aware of contractions in her womb, although these may be uncomfortable, they are very healthy and positive signs of the recovery of the woman's body after pregnancy.

The Oxytocin which stimulates uterine contractions also provides mild pain relief and enhances mood, as well as reinforcing the loving bond between mother and child, which can help to counteract any discomfort. These uterine contractions will only last as long as they are needed, for the first 40 days or so (often much less) and are therefore temporary, not a permanent part of breastfeeding your child. Hot water bottles (and other forms of gentle localized heat) can be very soothing to the discomfort of contractions, which can resemble menstrual cramps. If you are breastfeeding, you may wish to avoid taking Paracetamol or ibuprofen, although there are a variety of natural aromatherapy, homeopathy and naturopathic medicines available, which may be safe while lactating. Nutrition plays a vital role in providing the body with all the minerals and nutrients it needs to heal and repair optimally.

Oats are an excellent healthy (macrobiotic, vegan) source of nutritional support during the post-partum period, and even during menstruation, and offer the additional advantage of being a galactogen, which means that they help to promote and establish abundant milk flow in breastfeeding mothers. Oats can be consumed as hot porridge or baked in breads, cakes muffins, and flapjacks, as well as placed in smoothies dehydrated in cereal bars, or sprouted and made into oatmilk if you want to consume them raw. Integral oats have a much higher nutrient content than overly processed porridge oats, so be especially careful to consume wholegrain oats for the greatest benefits.

Cord Clamping

When the baby is born, it is still attached to the placenta via its umbilical cord, and it has been the custom within hospitals for many years to cut the cord immediately and remove the child from its mother for its first initial diagnostic tests. Cutting the cord quickly is considered necessary in some circumstances when artificial resuscitation must be given to the child (although limited research and anecdotal evidence suggest that these are the very circumstances in which the extra oxygenated blood received through the placenta can prevent the newborn from suffering brain damage and distress from asphyxiation).

Recent research has demonstrated the disadvantages to the child of cutting the cord too early, and many hospitals are now recognizing the advantages of delayed clamping. The World Health Organization now recommends delayed cord clamping wherever medically possible. Some hospitals recommend waiting three minutes after birth, although delayed clamping is recognized as being any time after one minute after the birth of the child. For full benefits, it is preferable to delay cord clamping until after the umbilical cord has stopped pulsing (which signifies that blood is no longer circulating through it).

While the pulsing (like a heartbeat) often finishes after the first three minutes (where the baby is kept level with the entrance to the mother's vagina), the pulsing of the cord can often continue up to 10 minutes after birth.

It is recommended that the umbilical cord be left intact and connected to the child at least until after it has finished pulsing. Under most conditions, a newborn will be able to reach its mother's breast while attached to the unborn placenta via the umbilical cord, and therefore it is unnecessary to cut the cord before the placenta is born. In some circumstances, the umbilical cord is too short, and it may be more critical for the mother to breastfeed her child and stimulate the birth of the placenta as soon as possible, so after the umbilical cord has stopped pulsing it can be clamped and cut to allow mobility for the child. The length of umbilical cord can vary between 40 and 70 cm.

The length of the umbilical cord is increased by the tension that the fetus produces on the cord while growing in the womb. A short cord is associated with a less active fetus, which may also coincide with fetal malformation, Down's syndrome, myopathies, neuropathies, and oligohydramnios. Short cords may result in rupture or hemorrhage.

Very long umbilical cords present their own dangers as there is a risk of the umbilical cord becoming looped or tied around the baby's neck or limbs or even being born before the baby. When an umbilical cord is born before the baby, (prolapse) it can become compressed. Since the umbilical cord supplies all the oxygen to the unborn child a compressed umbilical cord can cut off the baby's oxygen supply. A prolapsed umbilical cord is one of the increased risks of breech birth and multiple births and is a genuine emergency that warrants an emergency cesarean section being performed to save the life of the unborn child.

Nuchal cords (where the umbilical cord is wrapped around a baby's neck at birth, are surprisingly common "*Loosening the knot and unwrapping the tight coils from the neck and body is the first step of treatment. It is especially important in these cases that the cord not be cut, giving the placenta a chance to aid in the resuscitation of these baby's once blood flow through the cord is re-established.*" [2.]

The placenta is, during its time in the womb, an external organ of the child's body, and contains at any time roughly $^1/_3$ of the baby's blood flowing through it, this means that the blood in the placenta and umbilical cord is part of the baby's blood system. Delayed cord clamping does not increase a woman's blood loss. Once the baby is born, the umbilical cord will continue to pulse until all the blood from the placenta is returned to the child's body. The extra blood supplied through the umbilical cord to the child after birth is known as a placental transfusion. If the baby is not breathing when born, allowing the cord to continue pulsing means that the child will still receive oxygen through the cord, lowering the risk of problems related to oxygen starvation.

Delayed cord clamping has been observed to provide the following benefits for children: it decreases the risk of late-onset sepsis and necrotizing enterocolitis, it increases blood volume in the infant and reduces the need for blood transfusions caused by anemia or low blood pressure. In preterm children, it reduces the rates of inter-ventricular hemorrhage by up to 50%. It may also be of particular benefit to the neuro-development of male infants. Delayed cord clamping reduces the chance of a child having low ferritin levels (a protein in the blood which stores iron) and the benefits are long-term with children showing a reduced rate of anemia in studies up to the age of 3 years old.

Breastmilk contains all the nutrients, vitamins, minerals and calories that an infant requires. However, it does not provide iron, which is why babies are born with extra reserves of iron to last them until they are introduced to solid foods at around 4-6 months of age. Placental transfusion increases the level of iron in the body's system reducing the risk of anemia. Delayed umbilical cord clamping may be particularly relevant for infants living in low-resource settings with less access to iron-rich foods and thus, greater risk of anemia, this may also be a consideration for mothers who are vegan or vegetarian.

In some circumstances, health professionals have experimented with the technique of milking the umbilical cord, which means that they forcibly squeeze the content of the umbilical cord in the direction of the baby, in the effort to speed up the wait until the cord is cut. Milking the cord provides no discernible benefits and is not recommended as it is unnecessary and potentially harmful. Nature knows what it is doing, and until we can prove that we know better, we should not interfere.

Milking the cord may lead to discomfort, as the speed of absorption of the nutrients by the baby is increased, and it may prevent the flow of nutrients from the placenta into the umbilical cord. During the period after birth when the cord is pulsing there is an exchange of blood between the baby and the placenta, and blood can flow both ways. The baby will signal when it has received the right amount of blood and oxygen from the placenta, it cannot and should not be forced. Patience is a virtue.

"...in studies with monkeys, neurological disorders, memory, and behavioral defects were produced through cord camping. They did not occur in newborn monkeys that delivered without interference with the cord and placenta." [4.]

Delayed cord clamping may also be available during some cesarean births. So, if you are having a planned cesarean birth, it is wise to consider discussing delayed cord clamping and other sensitive practices as part of your birth plan. For those planning a vaginal birth, it may be worth drafting a backup cesarean birth plan, even if you intend never to use it. This emergency cesarean birth plan may be discussed with your Doula but should not necessarily be shown to the hospital or medical staff unless it becomes necessary to implement it. Having a backup cesarean plan available in the notes may persuade medical staff that they do not have to try so hard to accommodate your vaginal birth delivery wishes.

"The small or premature baby is much more vulnerable to injury from immediate cord clamping than the robust term child...if you find that you will need to deliver prematurely, you should impress upon the delivering physician the importance of letting the baby have its cord blood... neonatal units are filled with weak, fast-clamped newborns exhibiting signs of severe blood loss, pallor, hypovolemia (low blood volume) anemia (low blood count) hypotension (low blood pressure), hypothermia (cold), oliguria (poor urine output) metabolic acidosis, hypoxia (low oxygen supply) and respiratory distress (shock lung) to the point that some need blood transfusions and many more receive blood volume expanders," George Malcolm Morley, MD ChB, FACOG, How the cord Clamp in your baby's brain. .... When the cord is cut before the infant begins to breathe, the placental oxygen supply is instantly cut off, and the child remains asphyxiated until the lungs begin to function." [4]

"The energy that pulses through the cord from the placenta is the Divine Mother nourishing us. It is neither wholly our biological mother's nor ours"[1]

Jaundice

Anecdotal evidence suggests that children who have benefited from delayed cord clamping, may experience an increased likelihood of developing temporary jaundice after birth, this is due to the child possessing increased levels of blood in their system. Because children were deprived of the umbilical and placental blood for so long by hospital practices of early clamping, and because delayed cord clamping is a relatively new practice, many professionals are not aware of this potential connection.

Delayed cord clamping jaundice is caused by a build-up of excess bilirubin which must be processed by the liver. Adequate hydration (by breastfeeding on demand) and exposure to sunlight are often the only necessary treatments, and jaundice will clear up by itself within the first 2-3 weeks. However, some children born during winter months and those with darker skin (more melatonin protecting the skin from sunlight) are more likely to require additional exposure to sunlight than those with light skin or those born in the summer months when they are less bundled up and are naturally exposed to more natural light.

There are certain types of jaundice which can indicate life-threatening conditions, so it is always important to identify the cause of jaundice, and medical staff will monitor this condition carefully if it presents. It may be recommended that the child receive blood tests to definitively rule out any life-threatening conditions. However, since jaundice resulting from breastfeeding and jaundice which occurs in newborns due to having received their full share of cord blood, are both sensitive to phytotherapy; it may be worth requesting that your child be exposed to a special bilirubin light as a first step, before submitting them to blood tests to see if any positive results can be induced.

Newborn babies are very small they have a very small volume of blood. As a result, it is often necessary for medical staff to "milk" a child's wound to collect a sufficient blood sample for blood tests. This can be very uncomfortable and understandably traumatic for a newborn child, and may be contrary to the religious or ethical beliefs of the parents, so where possible non-invasive exposure to sunlight/ bilirubin lights would be my first choice. If, however, the child does not respond to phytotherapy it may be necessary to consider jaundice as a sign of a more dangerous illness. Parents can of course safely expose their children to sunlight by placing them naked or lightly covered by a sunny window in a warm place. Care should be taken to avoid chilling the child or letting it get sunburnt by exposure to very strong sunlight.

It is essential to make sure that the placenta is born intact, as a retained placenta can increase the risk of the mother developing an infection and fever. Although the placenta is usually round, some placentas grow with additional lobes, and it is important for medical staff to examine the placenta to ensure that there are no signs of the placenta being torn and pieces left within the womb. If the placenta is broken or becomes torn or detached from the umbilical cord, then it is vital that the umbilical cord be clamped immediately to prevent any chance of the baby bleeding out from this area. It is crucial that no one tries to encourage the birth of the placenta by pulling or tugging upon the umbilical cord from the outside as this increases the risk of tearing and retention of pieces of the placenta. In some severe circumstances, there have been reported incidents of uterine prolapse caused by medical staff pulling on the umbilical cord. Uterine prolapse is severe and life-threatening requiring surgery and can result in lifelong issues relating to subsequent fertility and continence, amongst other things.

If the placenta has not been born within the first hour, and the baby has already begun to breastfeed (which should stimulate uterine contractions), then it may be necessary to consider medical intervention such as a Pitocin injection. If Pitocin or any other synthetic Oxytocin injections are to be given to the mother, then it will be necessary to clamp and cut the baby's umbilical cord first.

Indications from "cord drainage" trials suggest that less blood-filled placentas shorten the third stage of labor and decreases the incidence of retained placenta and, therefore, increases the likelihood of the spontaneous birth of the placenta. This means delayed cord clamping increases the probability of the mother giving birth to the placenta intact without additional interventions.

"Ensuring placental completeness is of critical importance in the delivery room. Retained placental tissue is frequently associated with infection and hemorrhage. The fetal membranes need to be examined at the edges of the placenta. The prominence of vessels (large vessels) beyond the edges indicate that a placental lobe may have been retained (accessory lobe). All or part of the placenta is likely to be retained (in placenta accreta, placenta increta, and placenta percreta). ...A reduction in placental thickness, i.e., less than 2.5 cm is usually associated with intrauterine growth retardation of the fetus. When a placenta becomes thicker than normal, i.e., more than 4 cm in thickness, it is usually associated with fetal hydrops, maternal diabetes mellitus and intrauterine fetal infection (Fig 1.2).

Lotus Birth

The practice of lotus birth is relatively new but has become quite popular in peaceful-parenting circles. Lotus birth is where parents choose to keep the placenta with the child, and not cut the cord at all, instead, waiting for the cord to dry out and become detached as it would naturally and normally without intervention within the first week or so after the child is born.

The placenta is essentially raw flesh and left unfrozen and unrefrigerated for over a week it decomposes. Therefore parents use a variety of techniques such as salting (to dehydrate) the placenta as well as coating it with fresh herbs and essential oils to keep it from smelling bad or attracting insects. The placenta is usually kept in a small pouch that is carried around with the child, and parents and other caregivers must be very careful to avoid any pressure, tugging, or pulling on the cord during this time. The idea behind the lotus birth is that the delicate spirit of the child is sensitive to the cutting of the umbilical cord (its lifeline for 9 months and the physical manifestation of its connection to this plane of existence) and registers its severance as a shock, or a violence. Some consider this to be too traumatic for the newborn after having experienced the extreme turbulence of transitioning from the intrauterine environment of the mother to the outside world where it must breathe for itself.

While lotus birth is not a practice that has any historical or cultural precedence, some indigenous cultures recognize that the soul (or astral body) is attached to the physical body at the umbilicus. I have no personal experience with the lotus birth method. However, parents who are fans of this practice explain that they are easily able to care for their child while it is attached to the placenta, bathing their child with a sponge or washcloth rather than submerging the infant in water, which rehydrates the cord and prolongs its attachment.

"...chimpanzees immediately nurse their babies with the umbilical and placenta still attached, allowing the umbilical cord to dry up and separate without intervention, usually within a day of birth" [4.]

"Letting the placenta drop off and release by itself, usually between three to seven days after being born, leads to peace and the wisdom "I receive," "I have everything I need," [1.]

Ancient Traditions

The Navajo (or Denai, which is the name by which they refer to themselves) bury the umbilical cord of their children in the land so that no matter how far they roam on their journey of life, they will always return home.

"In many of the Plain's Tribes, the newborn was presented with a small beaded pouch that contained the remnants of their umbilical cord stump. The child would wear this throughout their lifetime, and many were buried with it in their old age. This talisman was thought to bring connectedness to the tribe, the individual family unit, and serve as protection. The Pueblo people would either bury the umbilical cord in the floor of the home (if it was a girl) or the cornfield (if it was a boy). On the fourth day after birth, the infant was presented to the sun, the shaman would name the child, and present the child with either an ear of corn (if it was a girl) or a flint arrowhead (if it was a boy)." [5.]

In some cultures, umbilical cords are dried and worn in charms and amulets, and they are considered so sacred and powerful that they must be protected from being stolen, as whoever holds the umbilical cord is believed to wield a magical influence upon the person and can make them do their bidding. Likewise, umbilical cords and dried placental tissue were often sought out for the casting of curses or love spells and oaths (such as marriage). The umbilical cord, is seen as the most sacred aspect linking not just to the person's life (and the umbilical cord as we can see is considered to have the power over life and death), but also to the eternal spirit of the individual which will continue after this body is gone.

Midwives traditionally helped with the ceremonial dedication or disposal of the umbilical cords, and placentas of the newborn babies that they delivered into their community. Having access to such important parts of the lives of so many of the community meant that the midwife had to be carefully chosen and extremely trustworthy.

In Europe during the middle ages, many midwives were portrayed as objects of fear for this very reason. They were perceived to have such power over life and death and were often imbued with extensive herbal and ceremonial knowledge that they would have the capacity to inflict great harm if they chose to.

It is not surprising that midwives were often persecuted as witches by the church who perceived a threat to their position of control and influence in the community. The witch trials also coincided with the birth of modern medicine. Alchemy (the precursor to Chemistry) and other sciences began to fall under the territory of the church, and many historians have remarked that our understanding of human biology was greatly advanced by the extensive implementation of torture by the Catholic Inquisition.

Of course, anything that could be used to harm could also be used to heal, and many midwives, herbalists, and healers also used the placental tissue and other identifying talismans to perform healing rituals and create fertility charms with the blessing of their community. The status that such people had in their community was very high, and a perceived threat to the churches complete control over the psyche of the population. By controlling the health of the population through control of the medical industry, their influence was enhanced.

Stem Cells

Umbilical cord blood and the placenta contain stem cells. Stem cells have the remarkable potential to develop into many different cell types in the body. Serving as a repair system for the body, they can theoretically divide without limit to replenish other cells if the person or animal is still alive. When a stem cell divides, each new cell has the potential to either remain a stem cell or to become another type of cell with a more specialized function, such as a muscle cell, a red blood cell, or a neuron. Stem cells are highly valued for medical research and for the treatment of various types of cancer and have the potential to be used in the treatment of Parkinson's disease, Alzheimer's, diabetes and any number of other debilitating, life-threatening and degenerative diseases.

Leukemia, Lymphoma, and Myeloma are three diseases that are commonly treated with stem cells, (in addition, a cancer suppressant substance called "Metastin" has been discovered in human placental tissue), and stem cells have also been used to treat blood disorders, congenital metabolic disorders, and immunodeficiencies.

Cord Blood Banking

Cord blood banking is a relatively new phenomenon that has developed to offer parents the opportunity to harvest stem cells from the umbilical blood of their children and store it for future use, as a potential medical back up for their child, or any other genetically compatible relatives such as a sibling.

Cord blood can be donated free of charge in the United States. However, cord blood banking for private use (saved explicitly for the infant or their family members) often requires a fee and an ongoing maintenance fee for the storage of the stem cells.

While the medical application of stem cells is potentially infinite, stem cell research is in its infancy, and there are no guarantees regarding when treatments will become available for specific illness and diseases. One of the most significant disadvantages of cord blood banking is the fact that delayed cord clamping, and cord blood banking are usually mutually exclusive.

Either your child gets the placental transfusion at the time of its birth, benefiting from its birthright immediately, or you harvest this blood and store it for a potential (hypothetical) use in the future.

The placenta is itself a plentiful source of stem cells. Traditionally stem cells have been harvested from the umbilical cords of newborn babies, bone marrow of children or adults, or aborted fetuses, or discarded test-tube embryos, although research is being done on developing techniques to harvest stem cells from menstrual blood and the placenta.

"...umbilical cord blood contains only small numbers of stem cells and extraction of bone marrow requires a painful needle and a very close match between donor and recipient to prevent rejection. Moreover, the use of embryos and fetal tissue as stem cell sources is extremely contentious."[6.]

"The topic of fetal tissue donation has come to light amid a series of videos released by the Center for Medical Progress, an anti-abortion group that accused Planned Parenthood of selling fetal tissue for-profit and of altering the way it performs abortions in order to gather more intact specimens." [7.]

"Hospitals used to sell placentas in bulk to drug and cosmetic companies, and for a while, doctors in burn wards used the membranes to cover large burned areas on their patients. But sometimes during the eighties, concerns about possible transmission of the AIDs virus and other contaminants largely put a stop to these practices." [2.]

" ...in the 1970s, Cuba exported 40 tons of human placentas to a French laboratory after discovering that it could be used to successfully treat vitiligo, a condition that causes the skin to lose pigment?" [8.]

Health and Beauty

In addition to medical research, the placenta is also used for a number of other purposes.

Human and animal placentas and placenta extracts are currently used in many cosmetics, pharmaceuticals and beauty products, with cosmetics including anti-aging creams, facials, hair conditioners, and controversial tonics and food products on the market.

Cleopatra and Marie Antoinette were both rumored to have used placentas in their beauty treatments. There was a great deal of rumor and accusation during European and Colonial American witch trials linking women (witches) with the consumption of and external use of placentas. Since most of the witches or wise women of the time also functioned as midwives, they would have been more likely to have access to placenta than the average layperson and may have been aware of its regenerative qualities.

Some midwives in developing countries recommend applying the placenta to the vagina shortly after birth to speed up the healing of any tearing or the wounds of an episiotomy, and on more than one occasion placentas have been applied as poultices to speed the healing of and encourage the healthy growth of tissue after surgery.

"Human placentas are also used by search and rescue teams to train their search and rescue dogs in human remains detection."[7.]

The remainder of human placentas abandoned at hospitals are often taken away and incinerated along with other "medical waste" like rubbish. This seems like a waste of a valuable resource considering that according to **Placenta Power: For Health and Beauty A useful guide for those seeking placenta-based remedies Kentaro Yoshida, Director of the Yoshida Clinic** the main medical functions of the placenta, or placental extract is as a treatment for: *Nervous System Regulatory Function (specifically the autonomous nervous system), Endocrine (Hormonal) System Regulatory Function, Immune System Function (raises resistance to illness), Basal Metabolism Function (energises the metabolism, activating cells, blood vessels and organs), Active Oxygen Removal Function (prevents oxidation), Anti-inflammatory Function, Tissue Repair Function, Tranquillising Function…. It has also been shown to have a number of other functions as follows; Anti-toxin Function (strengthens the liver), Lactation Promotion Function, Anti-Allergy Function, Constitution Function, Circulation Function, Blood Production Function, Anti-mutagen Function (suppresses mutations), Blood Pressure Regulatory Function, Fatigue Recovery Function, Appetite Promotion Function… Placenta Can Treat the Following Conditions Gynaecology: menopausal disorders, menstrual pain, irregular menstruation, failure of lactation, and high prolactin levels, etc. Internal Medicine: hepatitis, cirrhosis of the liver, chronic pancreatitis, diabetes, chronic gastritis, dyspepsia, gastric ulcers, duodenal ulcer, ulcerative colitis, bronchial asthma, chronic bronchitis, high blood pressure, low blood pressure, habitual constipation, and collagen disease, etc.*

Surgery: chronic rheumatoid arthritis, osteoarthritis, arthritis, neuralgia, lumbago, and stiff shoulders, etc. Dermatology: atopic skin complaints, psoriasis, body odor, eczema, chapped skin, spots, and freckles, etc. Psychiatry: autonomic ataxia, and sleeplessness, etc. Urology: enlarged prostate, cystitis, and hemorrhoids, etc. Ophthalmology: cataracts, allergic conjunctivitis, and vision loss, etc. Ear,

Nose, and Throat: allergic rhinitis, Meniere's disease, and hay fever, etc. Dentistry: pyorrhoea, and gum disease, etc. Other: fatigue, chills, weak constitution, recovery of strength during and after illness, muscularity, and strength of mind, etc."**9.**

Honoring the Placenta

There is a profound and sacred spiritual connection between the child and their placenta. Most indigenous cultures recognize this in one way or another through a ceremony which honors the placenta and the service that it has provided to the child.

The most common ceremony, found in a range of cultures throughout the world, is the burial of the placenta in a sacred space, often as a gift or offering to the Mother Earth and beneficial spirits, often commemorated and the location marked with the planting of a special tree or plant. The extraordinary nutritional value within the placenta provides a great resource to the growing plant, and many New Age and Spiritual westerners have adopted this ceremony of planting fruit trees to commemorate the burial of the placenta.

Certain superstitions surround these trees, since a sacred spiritual connection is said to link the child and the tree that was nourished by its Placenta. The health of the tree is said to be liked to the health of the child, felling of the tree, it is said, may kill the child, and for this reason, the tree needs to be protected and cared for as if it was the child. In some cultures, the location of the tree is kept secret in order to protect the child from malicious harm. In other cultures, the tree is planted close to the family home where it can be seen daily and where the child can maintain a relationship with it as it grows. Within these cultures moving or selling one's home would naturally be unthinkable, for the land has been made sacred.

In Jamaica, the children themselves are charged with the care of the tree. Their own spiritual link to its survival ensures their dedication and teaches the child responsibility and the interdependent relationship that all people have with the plants and trees within the environment. On a greater scale, it is worth observing that trees do indeed provide the oxygen and food that we depend upon in our environment and their survival is therefore intimately linked to our own.

Hospitals are required to return placentas to parents after they have been examined, provided that the parents make this request known.

Consuming the Placenta

There is another way that certain cultures honor the placenta and that it by consuming it. Either it is consumed by the mother to restore her nutrients and vital energies. Or rarely, the placenta is burnt in a ceremony with special herbs and the ashes fed to all members of the newborn's family or community, emphasizing the unity of the community in the shared responsibility of caring for that child, as a part of themselves.

Most mammals, do in fact, consume the placenta shortly after birth (including herbivores such as cows), and it is an anomaly that humans as a species do not. However, the tide may be turning in that regard.

Traditional Chinese Medicine has used dried human placenta in the treatment of numerous medical conditions for centuries. Modern women are beginning to consider the potential health benefits of placentophagy, with placenta encapsulation becoming more and more popular. There are even placenta recipe books available that suggest mixing dried placenta into homemade chocolates and adding raw placenta to fruit smoothies.

While the idea of consuming the placenta of another person seems dangerous and unethical, consuming the placental tissue which a mother generates herself may provide some advantages.

After giving birth, a woman's blood volume decreases drastically, and it is not uncommon for her to suffer from anemia, and low energy levels as her stores of iron and other vital nutrients are depleted.

The placenta is a rich source of easily digestible iron and other minerals including *"calcium, sodium, potassium, phosphorus, magnesium, and zinc,"* as well as vitamins *"B 1, B 2, B 6, B 12, C, D, E, and niacin.... The placenta has a history of medicinal use starting more than 2000 years ago. It was used as an elixir of eternal youth during the Qin Dynasty in China (259 BC to 210 BC)."* [9.]

Although many factors can contribute to post-partum depression, consumption of the placenta, and the unique combination of natural hormones and nutrients (specifically and genetically matched to the mother) that it can provide, has been cited as a beneficial treatment. Adequate nutrition is always an important factor in conserving the physical, mental, emotional and spiritual health of an individual, and nutrient deficiencies are well known to cause depressed mood and unbalanced mental states.

Placenta consumption is widely reported to elevate mood, restore hormonal balance, promote lactation and increase energy levels.

Dried placenta powder, (usually administered in the form of capsules) and placenta extract injections (now legally available in Japan), have been used in TCM for the treatment of a variety of conditions including: menopause, infertility, impotence, ulcers, psoriasis, eczema, arthritis, wasting diseases, uterine fibroids, endometriosis, mastitis, hepatitis, allergies, failure to lactate, and an astounding list of other ailments.

The placenta can be consumed raw, some people advocate freezing it in chunks and adding it to fresh fruits and nut milk and blending it into a daily smoothie or cooking it and eating it as you would a steak. `
Placenta encapsulation is popular, and you can usually find someone to provide this service for you, or even DIY it at home, all you really need is somewhere to cook the placenta, a dehydrator, and some empty capsules. Each placenta is reported to produce between 100-125 capsules. Women are encouraged to keep the capsules in the freezer and consume 2-3 per day (or as many as they feel they need) until the supply either runs out, or they don't want to take any more. Some women even store the capsules long term, for when they experience the onset of menopause and intend to use them as an alternative to hormone replacement therapy to gradually ease them through the process.

Of course, unless you have dozens of children the supply would run out quickly, which is why animal placentas and human placenta extract injections are offered as alternatives. Placenta capsules are also reported to be useful in treating menstrual discomfort. Once regular menstrual cycles return, some women may wish to save their capsules for these future events if they have a history of painful periods.

Traditional placenta encapsulation follows the TCM method of cooking the placenta prior to dehydration, although some raw foodists are advocating dehydrating raw placenta for encapsulation instead. They argue that many of the nutrients and hormones are degraded through the cooking process and that the heat destroys the enzymes.

Whenever meat is dried for consumption without cooking or smoking it first, such as in the case of some jerky, it is heavily coated is salt, (sometimes nitrate), herbs, spices, and other ingredients to prevent bacterial colonization, and maintain its safety for consumption. If you encapsulate your placenta raw, it would either have a very short shelf life (possibly extended if stored frozen) or it would need to be adulterated with other substances such as high levels of salt (a natural preservative), cayenne pepper and other antiparasitics. Taking high levels of salt daily is not a good idea, and you would need to consider the effect that any of the other ingredients might have on your body before self-medicating with them.

Another potential use for the placenta is to make a tincture from it using 100+ proof alcohol (such as vodka). A small piece of placenta is submerged into alcohol and left to cure for up to 6 weeks, the alcohol is then strained, and the resulting tincture is referred to as the mother tincture. From this mother tincture, it is possible to make a tincture that is ready to consume by diluting about 30 drops of the other tincture with 1 oz of half water and half alcohol mixture. This produces a higher quantity of medicine than encapsulation, and the tincture may last for years. I have no data on the effectiveness of this form of treatment, however since it only requires a small piece of the placenta you may wish to try it in addition to encapsulation for when the capsules run out and compare any differences that you perceive.

You could also turn your placenta into a variety of creams, ointments and beauty products, or try applying it directly to your face as a facial instead of investing large sums of money on professional masks containing sheep placenta stem cells which are reported to rejuvenate the skin, improve skin tone and boost collagen.

You may have to fight for you right to retain your placenta if you are having a hospital birth. In certain circumstances, doctors would prefer to send the placenta to pathology to be tested, and this may become necessary if meconium was detected during labor. However, only a small portion of the placenta is usually required (no bigger than the size of an egg at most), and it may be possible for you to take the rest of the placenta home if you want to use it for encapsulation, etc. If you intend to honor the placenta through ceremony, it may be contradictory to your beliefs to allow a portion of the placenta to be separated from the whole. Make sure if you intend to consume the placenta that it is not injected with formaldchyde or any other dangerous toxins.

Honouring the placenta has become common practice over the last few years, and artists have come up with many creative ways to preserve the placenta and umbilical cord as mystical keepsakes and talismans. One example of this is the placenta drum made from the membrane which covers the placenta. Another is a dream-catcher, where the outer ring is made from the umbilical cord dried in the shape of a hoop or circle.

Conclusion

The humble placenta has been gravely overlooked and undervalued for too long. It is time that we seriously considered taking better care of these fleshy guardians and requesting their return. Whether you choose to use the placenta as a medicine, a beauty treatment, a dietary supplement or plant fertilizer for your garden, or if you intend to find your own way of honoring your child's "twin soul" you can certainly find a better home for it than designating it to medical waste. For all that the placenta does for us and our children, healing, protecting and nurturing their young lives. The placenta deserves our gratitude and respect. I wish you good use.

Blessings

Bibliography

1. Womb Wisdom: Awakening the Creative and Forgotten Powers of the Feminine by Padma Aon Prakasha, Anaiya Aon Prakasha

2. Midwife: A Calling (Memoirs of an Urban Midwife) (Volume 1), by Peggy Vincent, RN, CNM.

3. Wise Woman Herbal for the Childbearing Years by Susan Weed.

4. The nourishing traditions book of baby and child care by Sally Fallon Morell, Thomas S. Cowan

5. Bellies and Baby's; A Sacred Journey by Nicole D http://wonderfullymadebelliesandbaby's.blogspot.cl/2010/11/sacred-journey.html

6. Placental stem cells The Royal Women's Hospital website.

7. Alternative uses for placenta From Wikipedia, the free encyclopedia

8. Placenta: The Gift of Life. Cornelia Enning, Author; Cheryl K. Smith, Editor. 2007. Motherbaby Press.

9. Placenta Power: For Health and Beauty A useful guide for those seeking placenta-based remedies Kentaro Yoshida, Director of the Yoshida Clinic

Did you enjoy this book?
Would you like to read more from
Jemmais Keval-Baxter
The Ho'oponopono Doula™?

Visit: www.hooponoponodoula.com
sign up for the mailing list to receive Free
resources and information about workshops,
books, services and events.

Other books in the series include:
A Doulas Guide to Education
A Doulas Guide to Nutrition
A Doulas Guide to Breastfeeding
A Doulas Guide to Menstruation

Also by Jemmais Keval-Baxter
Ho'oponopono Birth: Ho'oponopono for
Pregnancy and Childbirth.

If you liked this book, please leave a review so
that others can find it too.

About the Author

*Mrs. Jemmais Keval-Baxter resides in Chile with her family. She is a Natural Childbirth Coach, Doula, Doula Trainer, Writer, and EFT Coach. For more information about her books and workshops, please consult her website at **www.hooponoponodoula.com**.*

www.ingramcontent.com/pod-product-compliance
Lightning Source LLC
Chambersburg PA
CBHW060703280326
41933CB00012B/2282